The Nourishing Healing Elixir

The Remarkable Benefits
of
Castor Oil Unleashed

Maggie D. Keck

Copyright ©

Retained without approval from the publisher or creator.

TABLE OF CONTENT

Safety precautions

In summary

INTRODUCTION

The Ancient Elixir

Few substances have a more illustrious history in natural treatments than castor oil. This golden, viscous liquid derived from the humble castor bean has endured millennia, establishing its position in the pantheon of traditional medicines.

Discover the rich history.

Castor oil's origins can be traced back to ancient Egypt, when it was first recorded in the Ebers Papyrus, one of the world's oldest medical writings. It was a pharaoh's ally against illness and was revered for its purgative properties. The oil spread to the bazaars of Rome and Greece, where it was traded as a skin treatment and lamp fuel, illuminating the wisdom of professors and sages.

Castor oil made its way into Ayurvedic procedures in India throughout the years, where it was used with herbs to balance the body's humors. Healers in the Americas accepted it because of its great anti-inflammatory and antibacterial effects.

Today, we stand on the shoulders of these ancient traditions, while contemporary science begins to solve the riddles that our forefathers perceived. Castor oil, once a healer's secret, today makes its healing touch available to anybody seeking the knowledge of nature's elixir.

Embark on this trip through time to see how castor oil has cured, calmed, and enhanced people's lives, emerging as a beacon of natural healing in a world constantly seeking well-being.

Chapter 1

The Science of Castor Oil: Unlocking Nature's Healing Elixir

Castor Bean: A Botanical Marvel.

Before we go into the complex chemistry of castor oil, let us first honor its modest source: the castor bean (*Ricinus communis*). This modest seed, native to Africa and India, has a wealth of healing potential beneath its thick shell. Its botanical history spans thousands of years, mingling with human civilization, folklore, and medicine.

Castor Beans Chemical Symphony

1. **Ricinoleic Acid**: The Leading Player
- Castor oil contains ricinoleic acid, which is its secret weapon. This unsaturated fatty acid, which accounts for almost **90%** of the oil, follows its rhythm. Its unusual

structure—a hydroxy group connected to a double bond—gives it exceptional characteristics. Ricinoleic acid acts as a **hydrophilic** and **lipophilic** molecule, bridging the gap between water and oil. This dual attraction enables it to easily penetrate skin, hair, and membranes, delivering its therapeutic payload.

2. **Hydroxy Fatty Acids**: Allies for Wellness

- Aside from ricinoleic acid, castor oil contains additional hydroxy fatty acids. These are **dihydroxystearic acid**, **hydroxystearic acid**, and **ricinoleic acid**. Their presence increases castor oil's viscosity, making it thick and sticky—a physical reminder of its potency.

3. **Triglycerides**: Molecular Carriers.
- Castor oil is made up primarily of triglycerides, three fatty acid

chains connected to a glycerol backbone. These molecular trios transport ricinoleic acid to its intended locations within the body. They move through cell membranes, sebaceous glands, and hair follicles, ensuring the elixir's enchantment reaches every nook and cranny.

The Healing Symphony: Castor Oil Properties

☐ Anti-inflammatory Maestro**

- Ricinoleic acid leads to an anti-inflammatory symphony. It soothes sensitive skin, reduces redness, and relieves joint discomfort. Castor oil's anti-inflammatory properties are particularly effective when applied to inflamed acne or massaged into tight muscles.

☐ Lubricant and Barrier Composer**.
- Castor oil's viscosity forms a protective barrier. It protects

fragile tissues, retains hydration, and reduces water loss. From chapped lips to cracked heels, this natural emollient meets our skin's demands.

 The Detox Conductor**
- When consumed, castor oil exerts a detoxifying effect. It stimulates the intestines and encourages them to discharge toxins. Ancient healers valued it as a purgative that cleansed both body and spirit.

☐ Hair Growth Virtuosa**

- The hydroxy fatty acids serenade the hair follicles, stimulating growth. Castor oil's nurturing cadence strengthens strands, prevents breakage, and reactivates latent follicles. A scalp massage with this elixir creates a symphony of healthy locks.

☐ The Immune System Harmonizer**

- Castor oil's diverse makeup works well with our immune

system. It regulates immunological responses and promotes equilibrium. It orchestrates immunity's delicate dance, just like a trained conductor would.

Unleashing the Elixir's Potential

As we untangle the castor bean's chemical symphony, we can see the exquisite soundtrack that has resonated throughout civilizations. Castor oil has been used by pharaohs in ancient Egypt and Ayurvedic sages to treat various ailments. Today, armed with scientific knowledge, we respect this elixir—nature's everlasting gift.

Chapter 2

Skin and Hair Health: Castor Oil's Transformative Magic

Castor oil, with its rich content, transforms into a nourishing elixir for the skin. Nourishing your skin while increasing radiance and hydration. This is how it performs its magic:

Deep Moisturization: Castor oil penetrates deeply, providing moisture to dry skin. Massage a few drops onto your face, hands, or other dry areas, and watch as your skin's need is quenched.

Anti-Aging Properties: The fatty acids in castor oil, particularly **ricinoleic acid**, promote collagen formation. Collagen, the skin's structural protein, prevents wrinkles and preserves flexibility. Regular use can help you defy time's hold.

Healing Blemishes: Castor oil heals acne scars, stretch marks, and small wounds. Its anti-inflammatory qualities calm sensitive skin, and its antioxidants aid in tissue healing.

1. Unlocking Lustrous Hair and Hair Growth.

- **Root Awakening**: Castor oil nourishes hair follicles and stimulates dormant ones. Apply it to your scalp, massage it gently, and let it promote hair development. Say welcome to thicker, fuller hair.

- **Minimising Hair Loss**: Ricinoleic acid included in castor oil strengthens hair shafts, minimizing breaking. Say goodbye to excessive shedding and welcome a healthier mane.

- **Soothing Scalp Inflammation**: If you suffer from dandruff or itchy scalp, castor oil's anti-inflammatory properties can help. It alleviates irritation, regulates sebum production, and leaves your scalp in harmony.

- **Lustrous Shine**: Apply a few drops of castor oil to the ends of your hair to transform dullness into shine. It binds split ends, reduces frizz, and adds a natural luster.

2. Ritual of Application and Warm Embrace

- **Warm It Up**: Before using, warm the oil slightly. This improves its absorption and provides a delightful sensation.

- **Massage Ritual**: Gently massage the oil into your skin or scalp. Circular motion promotes circulation and amplifies its effects.

- **Overnight Magic**: For an extensive treatment, apply castor oil overnight. Cover your hair with a shower hat and wrap your skin in a soft cloth. Wake up with regenerated skin and hair.

3. Safety Notes and Patch Test Prelude

- **Patch Test**: Always run a patch test before launching the entire application. Apply a little amount to a discrete place (such as your inner arm) and watch for any unpleasant effects.

- **Eye Caution**: Avoid making direct contact with the eyes. If this occurs accidentally, thoroughly rinsed with water.

Chapter 3

Beneficial Effects of Castor Oil on Digestive Health

The Interesting Role of Castor Oil

The digestive system plays a crucial role in our bodies' complicated theater. It orchestrates the conversion of food into energy, nutrients, and waste, creating a symphony of enzymes, acids, and peristaltic waves. Among this spectacular spectacle, castor oil emerges as a backstage magician, quietly casting healing charms.

Castor Oil Elixir is a gentle laxative

When consumed, castor oil takes on a dual role: it acts as an emollient as well as a stimulant. Let us look at its diverse role in promoting digestive wellness:

1. **Lubricating the GI Tract**
- The viscosity of castor oil covers the intestinal lining, allowing stool

to move more easily. It whispers to the bowels to encourage smooth flow. When constipation strikes, castor oil lends a kind hand.

2. **Stimulating peristalsis**
- The heartbeat of digestion is peristalsis, or the rhythmic contraction of the intestines. Castor oil stirs it awake. Ricinoleic acid harmonizes with gastrointestinal receptors, encouraging them to dance. What

was the result? A choreography of elimination.

3. **Detoxify the Liver and Gallbladder**
- Castor oil has a positive effect on our metabolic maestro, the liver. It increases bile flow, facilitating digestion and detoxifying. Castor oil stimulates gallbladder contractions, ensuring a consistent flow of bile.

4. **Balancing gut microbes**

- A thriving microbial colony exists beneath the mucosal membrane. Castor oil, with its antibacterial properties, preserves homeostasis. It reduces inflammation, controls unruly bacteria, and promotes healthy gut flora.

Castor Oil Ritual to Promote Digestive Harmony

Morning Elixir - Rise with the sun and drink your castor oil elixir. A teaspoonful, possibly, combined with warm water or herbal tea. Allow it to welcome your intestines like a peaceful daybreak.

Patience and Timing
- Castor oil's magic works gradually. Give it time. Avoid ingesting it before bedtime because it prefers daylight for dance.

Hydration Symphony

- Castor oil's lubricating properties flourish in a properly hydrated body. Drink water throughout the day to allow it to mingle perfectly with the elixir.

Safety Notes

Moderation Matters
- Castor oil is extremely potent. A little goes a long way. Overindulgence may cause cramping and pain.

Individual variations

- Our bodies waltz to different rhythms. Some people are eager to use castor oil, while others are hesitant. Listen to your body's whispers.

Consultation Prelude

- If you have a chronic ailment or are taking medications, consult with your doctor.

Chapter 4

Detoxing and cleansing

Castor Oil's Purification Journey

**1. **The Quest for Detoxification

Toxins lurk in the bustling maze of our bodies, unwelcome guests of our modern lifestyles. They creep in through dirty air, processed foods, and hectic days. Our organs—the liver, kidneys, and intestines—bear the brunt of this quiet invasion. Enter castor oil, the ancient sentinel with cleansing abilities.

Castor Oil Elixir: A Cleansing Symphony

1. **Liver Love Affair**
- Our liver, the tireless alchemist, converts poisons into safe chemicals. Castor oil provides stimulation to this crucial organ. It increases bile flow, encouraging the liver to release accumulated poisons. Bile cascades from the

gallbladder like a purifying waterfall.

2. **Internal Sweep**
- The viscosity of castor oil coats the intestinal walls, much like a gentle broom. It nudges stagnant waste, collected debris, and undigested remains. Peristalsis, the gut's rhythmic contractions, becomes active. The bowels, grateful, discharge their contents. Constipation disappears, replaced by a sense of lightness.

3. **Lymphatic flow**

- Our lymphatic system, like a silent river, transports immune cells and trash. Castor oil massages the currents. It reduces swelling in the lymph nodes, promotes lymph flow, and communicates with the immune system. Detoxification turns into a harmonious ballet.

4. **Cellular rejuvenation**

- The mitochondria, or life-giving powerhouses, hum within our cells. Castor oil, which contains ricinoleic acid, nourishes these little dynamos. It boosts cellular vitality, helping cells to cleanse properly. The body's symphony performs a renewed music.

Ritual of Castor Oil Detox

1. *The Elixir*
- Take one teaspoon of castor oil every morning. Combine it with warm water or herbal tea. Allow it

to run through your digestive system, washing away stagnation. Patience is its partner; the consequences come gradually.

2. *Abdominal Massage**
- Warm the oil between your palms. Gently rub your abdomen in clockwise circles. Visualize it reaching every nook and cranny, including the liver, intestines, and lymph nodes. Your touch becomes a purifying ritual.

3. **Hydratory Symphony**
- Castor oil flourishes in a well-hydrated environment. Drink water throughout the day. Imagine it merging with the elixir, boosting the cleansing effects.

 **Safety Notes

1. **Moderate and Respect**
- Castor oil is extremely potent. Respect its strength. Excessive doses should be avoided as they may cause discomfort.

2. **Individual Tempo**

- Pay attention to your body's tempo. Some dance quickly with castor oil, while others waltz cautiously. Respect your rhythm.

3. **Consultation Prelude**

- If you have any health notes or prescriptions, visit your healthcare conductor. They will lead your detox symphony.

Chapter 5

Anti-inflammatory Maestro

Castor oil has been shown to help reduce pain and inflammation. Ricinoleic acid, the star of castor oil's chemical symphony, is responsible for its anti-inflammatory properties. When administered topically, castor oil creates a calming effect:

- **Joint Pain**: Castor oil's mild massage will help relieve arthritis, painful muscles, and stiff joints. Its anti-inflammatory properties reduce inflammation and allow joints to move more easily.

- **Skin Inflammation**: Castor oil soothes sunburns and insect bites like a refreshing breeze. It decreases redness, alleviates irritation, and improves skin healing. Apply freely to inflamed areas and allow the harmonizing combination to perform its magic.

Castor Oil Packs: A Ritual for Relief

Castor oil packs**, a time-honored custom, allows you to participate in a healing ritual. Here's how you can compose your peaceful symphony:

 Materials Required

- **Organic Castor Oil**: Use cold-pressed, hexane-free castor oil.
- **Flannel Cloth or Cotton Fabric**: Wide enough to cover the damaged area.

- **Hot Water Bottle or Heating Pad**: To provide mild warmth.

**Application Steps

- **Soak the Fabric**: Soak the fabric in heated castor oil until well saturated.

- **Place on Skin**: Apply the oil-soaked cloth to the uncomfortable or irritated area.

- **Warm Embrace**: Place a hot water bottle or heating pad on top of the cloth. The warmth improves absorption.

- **Relax and Rest**: Lie down, close your eyes, and let the castor oil's healing vibrations penetrate your body. Inhale deeply.

**duration and frequency

- Leave the castor oil pack on for **30 minutes to an hour**.
- Repeat this ritual **2 to 3 times each week** for long-lasting relief.

**Safety Notes

- **Patch Test Prelude**: Always perform a patch test before using castor oil widely. Apply a tiny amount to a discreet place and watch for any unwanted responses.
- **Consultation Prelude**: If you have a chronic ailment or are using drugs, please consult your healthcare conductor. They will lead your pain-relief symphony.

Chapter 6

Castor Oil and Reproductive Wellness

What is castor oil?

Castor oil, extracted from the seeds of the *Ricinus communis* The plant has a long history dating back thousands of years. It was used by the Egyptians for oil lamps, and its moisturizing characteristics make it a popular ingredient in skincare products today. Aside from cosmetics, castor oil has a fascinating range of advantages, including the possible impact on reproductive health.

 Castor Oil Pack: A Healing Ritual
A **castor oil pack** is a wool flannel soaked in castor oil and applied to certain parts of the body. Let's look at how it can favorably impact reproductive health:

1. Castor oil packs improve blood circulation to reproductive organs, including the uterus, ovaries, and fallopian tubes. Fresh, oxygen-rich blood nourishes these essential reproductive organs, allowing them to function optimally.

2. **Reduced Inflammation and Pain**. Castor oil packs might help relieve uncomfortable periods or cramps. Their anti-inflammatory qualities reduce discomfort and

make menstrual cycles more bearable.

3. **Liver Detoxification** - A healthy liver promotes hormonal balance. Castor oil packs, when administered to the liver, aid in detoxification. Remember that a healthy liver promotes overall reproductive health.

4. **Stimulated Lymphatic System**. The lymphatic system lacks a pump (unlike the

circulatory system). Castor oil packs promote lymph circulation and waste clearance. In doing so, they indirectly support immunological activity.

A Simple Guide for Using Castor Oil Packs

1. **Materials Required**: - A hot water bottle.
- Wool flannel (made specifically for castor oil packs).

- Plastic sheet (to cover the package)

- Organic, cold-pressed castor oil.

- Old clothes and linens with castor oil stains!

2. **Application Steps**: Soak the wool flannel in castor oil.

- Apply it to the desired location (e.g., lower abdomen for fertility, liver for detox).

- Use a hot water bottle to provide mild warmth.

- Relax and let the healing process take its course.

3. **Frequency**: - Apply castor oil packs for an hour to an hour and a half, 4 times a week for at least 3 months.

- Increase the frequency throughout your ovulation cycle if you are actively trying to conceive.

Safety precautions

1. **Patch Test**: Always run a patch test before extensive use.

2. **Consultation**: If you have any specific health concerns, speak with a healthcare practitioner.

Chapter 7

Castor Oil and Your Immune System

Castor oil, made from the seeds of the *Ricinus communis* The plant has been used for millennia because of its health benefits. Among its numerous benefits, castor oil is well known for its ability to boost the immune system. Here's a detailed look at how castor oil can help enhance immunity:

1. Lymphatic System Support

The lymphatic system is an important aspect of the immune system. It generates and transports lymphocytes, which are white blood cells that combat infection. Castor oil may promote lymphatic circulation, leading to increased immune cell formation and activity.

2. Thymus Gland Activation

The thymus gland is another important immunological organ that generates T-cells, a kind of lymphocyte that protects the body from invaders. Applying castor oil packs to the body may increase thymus gland function and boost immunological response.

3. Anti-inflammatory properties
Inflammation is a normal immunological response, but persistent inflammation can cause a variety of health problems.

Castor oil contains ricinoleic acid, which has anti-inflammatory effects that can reduce inflammation and improve immunological function.

4. Antimicrobial effects
Castor oil includes chemicals with antibacterial activity. These can aid the body in fighting illnesses by limiting the growth of bacteria, viruses, yeasts, and molds. This preventive action is especially good for the epidermis, the body's

first line of defense against external pathogens.

5.Detoxification
Castor oil can help with the body's natural detoxification processes by boosting the lymphatic and liver systems. Toxin removal can improve immune system performance by reducing its burden.

6.Maintaining Digestive Health

The gut contains a large element of the immune system. Castor oil can assist in maintaining a healthy digestive tract, which in turn promotes a strong immune system. It promotes healthy bowel movements and balances gut flora.

7.Antioxidant Content
Castor oil contains a high concentration of antioxidants, which are molecules that protect cells from free radical damage.

Antioxidants can protect immune cells from oxidative stress, which can decrease the immunological response.

 Using Castor Oil to Improve Immune Health

Castor Oil Packs

One of the most effective ways to use castor oil for immune support is to apply it in the form of packs. These entail soaking a cloth in castor oil and applying it to the skin, usually with heat, to improve absorption. This approach promotes lymphatic drainage and enhances immunological function.

Topical Application
Applying castor oil straight to the skin can help combat skin infections and enhance the skin's immune function. Massage it into joints and muscles to reduce inflammation and pain, potentially improving immunological health.

Oral consumption

While less frequent, certain traditional methods recommend ingesting castor oil orally to improve immunological function. However, due to its strong laxative effects, oral administration should be done with caution and under the supervision of a healthcare professional.

Safety Consideration
Castor oil offers numerous potential benefits for

immunological health, but it's crucial to use it responsibly.

- Always conduct a patch test before using castor oil extensively to ensure that you do not have an allergic reaction.
- Before using castor oil, see a healthcare expert, especially if you have any underlying health concerns or are pregnant.
- For optimal performance and safety, use high-quality, cold-

pressed castor oil that is free of hexane.

Finally, castor oil can be an effective strategy for improving immunological function. Its capacity to assist the lymphatic system, reduce inflammation, and fight off pathogens makes it an important component of a holistic approach to wellness.

Chapter 8

Castor Oil as a Mind Soother.

Castor oil, while historically renowned for its physical health advantages, also has benefits for mental and emotional wellness. Here's a detailed look at how castor oil might benefit the mind and emotions:

1.Stimulating the Parasympathetic Nervous System.

The parasympathetic nervous system is sometimes referred to as the "rest and digest" system. It helps to balance the body's stress reaction. Castor oil packs have been demonstrated to enhance relaxation by stimulating this system. This can help relieve tension and anxiety.

2. Promoting Relaxation and Sleep

Castor oil provides substantial benefits, including improved sleep. Castor oil might help you sleep better by lowering stress and boosting relaxation. Getting enough sleep promotes emotional resilience and mental clarity.

3. Supporting the Emotional Transition During Menopause

Menopause can be a difficult emotional and psychological transition. Castor oil, when used in aromatherapy or as part of a relaxation practice, can provide a calming effect. This can help manage stress and promote overall well-being during transitions.

4. Relieving Symptoms of Chronic Stress

Chronic stress can affect almost every bodily function. Using a castor oil pack can alleviate symptoms including inflammation, digestive difficulties, and stomach pain, allowing the body to recover from the effects of stress. Resting with a castor oil pack allows for deeper respiration and relaxation.

5. Detoxification Effects on Emotional Health

Castor oil's detoxifying properties extend beyond the physical realm. Castor oil helps remove pollutants and promotes emotional balance and well-being.

6. Developing Holistic Self-Care Practices

Castor oil can help people feel more empowered and in charge of their health. This can lead to increased self-esteem and a more hopeful outlook on life.

Using a castor oil pack is laying a cloth soaked in castor oil on the skin, frequently with heat to improve absorption. This practice is effective for soothing the mind and body.

Topical Application
Massaging castor oil into your skin will also produce a relaxing sensation. The massage itself is relaxing and can help reduce tension and anxiety.

Aromatherapy

The fragrance of castor oil can be used in aromatherapy to create a calming environment. The mild smell might help to soothe the mind and enhance the mood.

**Safety Consideration

Castor oil offers numerous potential benefits for emotional health, but it's vital to use it responsibly.

- Always conduct a patch test before using castor oil extensively to ensure that you do not have an allergic reaction.

- Before using castor oil, see a healthcare expert, especially if you have any underlying health concerns or are pregnant.

Finally, castor oil can be an effective supplement to emotional health practices. Its ability to promote relaxation, increase sleep, and support the body during stress makes it a useful tool for achieving mental and emotional well-being.

Chapter 9

Practical Applications of Castor Oil.

Castor oil, a versatile vegetable oil, has been utilized for thousands of years for its therapeutic properties. Here's how you can integrate it into your everyday routine and what safety precautions you should take:

1. Skin Care** - *Moisturiser*: Apply castor oil to dry skin to

moisturize and encourage healthy skin.

- **Cleaner**: Use as a natural cleanser to eliminate pollutants and improve your complexion.

2. Hair Care** - Scalp Treatment**: Massage castor oil into your scalp to promote hair development and prevent dandruff.

- **hair conditioner**: Apply evenly throughout your hair for deep conditioning and shine.

3.   Digestive   Health** -
Constipation Relief: Use a tiny quantity of castor oil as a stimulant laxative on an infrequent basis.

4. Joint and Muscle Health - **Pain Relief**: Apply castor oil to painful joints or muscles to lessen pain and inflammation.

5.   Immune   System   Support: **Castor Oil Packs**. To promote lymphatic   drainage   and

immunological function, place a castor oil-soaked cloth and a heating pad over the abdomen.

6. Holistic Practices** - **Stress Reduction**: Include castor oil packs in your relaxation practice to relieve stress and promote calm.

Safety precautions

1. Patch Testing- Before using castor oil on sensitive skin,

perform a patch test to prevent allergic reactions.

2. Excessive usage of castor oil, a potent laxative, can cause cramps, diarrhea, and digestive issues.

3. Pregnancy and Menstruation** - Women who are pregnant, menstruating, or trying to conceive should avoid putting castor oil packs on their abdomens.

4. Eye Contact** - Keep castor oil away from the eyes to avoid irritation.

5. Open Flames** - Castor oil is combustible, therefore keeping it away from open flames and heat sources.

6. Fabric Stains** - Castor oil can stain fabrics and, therefore, apply with old towels or clothes.

7. Medical Consultation**: Seek advice from a healthcare expert before taking castor oil for medical purposes, especially if you have underlying health conditions.

Incorporating castor oil into your daily regimen can provide several benefits, including improved skin and hair health and digestive assistance. However, it is critical to use it carefully and be mindful of its strong effects. By following these practical guidelines and safety precautions, you can safely enjoy the many benefits of this ancient elixir.

In summary

Castor oil is a flexible elixir that provides numerous benefits. Let us recap:

1. **Skin and Hair Health**: Castor oil moisturizes, stimulates hair development, and alleviates inflammation.
2. **Digestive Wellness**: It promotes proper digestion,

stimulates peristalsis, and aids in detoxifying.

3.   **Detoxification and Cleansing**: Castor oil aids liver detoxification, regulates gut bacteria, and cleanses the body.

4.   **Pain Relief and Inflammation**: It alleviates pain, lowers joint discomfort, and soothes skin inflammation.

5. **Fertility and Reproductive Health**: Castor oil packs can increase blood flow to the reproductive organs.

6. **Boosting Immunity**: It promotes the lymphatic system, balances gut health, and contains antioxidants.

7. **Mind and Emotions**: Castor oil promotes relaxation, improves sleep, and aids with emotional transitions.

8. **Practical Applications and Safety**: Apply castor oil packs, massage, and aromatherapy. Always patch tests and speak with an expert.

Incorporate this ancient elixir into your daily routine with care, and let its healing properties develop.

www.ingramcontent.com/pod-product-compliance
Lightning Source LLC
Chambersburg PA
CBHW050821250726

48653CB00006B/2352